WIN OVER DEPRESSION AND ANXIETY:

GREAT TIPS TO OVERCOME WORRY, FEAR, STRESS, PANIC ATTACKS, CONTROL EMOTIONS, DEVELOP EMOTIONAL INTELLIGENCE AND IMPROVE RELATIONSHIPS AFTER COVID 19 WITH SELF HELP, MEDITATION, EXERCISE, NATURE, LAUGH, FRIENDS AND FAMILY

Table of Contents

Introduction

Depression

Depression is a terrible feeling that comes to you from nowhere. A sensation you can't quite shake. As some would say you do, it's never as easy as "just snap out of it" Look, it's not easy, I know. Life's rough. I know. But it's your duty to attempt to defeat this ghost. To conquer everything thrown at you, you have got everything you need. It will take some time. But soon, you'll see the sun.

One of the most common mental health conditions in the world is depression. Although most people think depression is simply a condition itself, it is more specifically an umbrella for many more complex conditions, many of which are labeled depressive. They are more likely to speak about dysthymia, a moderate but chronic long-term depressive symptom, or major depressive disorder, including intense periods of depression. In contrast, most individuals claim they suffer from depression.

Depression is misunderstood and misdiagnosed widely. It's mixed up with stress. And, if you've never experienced major depression or seen anyone else go through it yourself, it's always hard to realize.

Symptoms and Signs of Depression

It can get worse and last for months, even years, if the depression goes untreated. As it does for around 1 out of 10 people with depression, it can cause discomfort and potentially lead to suicide.

It's essential to understand the signs. Sadly, almost half of individuals who have depression never get it diagnosed or treated.

It can contain the following symptoms:

- Tiredness

- Digestive disorders that are not getting better, even with medication

• Feelings of remorse, sense of worthlessness

• Insomnia, early-morning wakefulness, or too much sleep

• Irritability

• Difficulties in focusing, recalling facts, and making decisions

• Restlessness

• Loss of interest in once pleasurable activities, like sex

• Pessimism and hopelessness

• Overeating, or lack of appetite

• Aches, nausea, headaches, or cramps that will not go anywhere

• Persistent feelings that are sad, nervous, or "empty."

• Suicidal ideas or attempts

Types of Depression

Mild and moderate depression

The most popular kinds of depression are mild and moderate depression. The symptoms associated with mild depression can affect your everyday life more than just feeling blue, robbing you of joy and motivation. In moderate depression, those symptoms are exacerbated and can lead to a loss of trust and self-esteem.

Major depression

Major depression, characterized by severe, relentless symptoms, is often less common than mild or moderate depression.

Atypical depression

Atypical depression, with a particular symptom pattern, is a common subtype of major depression. It responds better than others to specific treatments and drugs, so it can help recognize it.

Seasonal affective disorder (SAD)

In certain individuals, decreased winter daylight hours contribute to a type of depression known as seasonal affective disorder (SAD). Around 1 percent to 2 percent of the population is affected by SAD, particularly women and young people. SAD can make you feel like a person different from who you are in the summer: helpless, sad, nervous, or anxious, without any interest in friends or activities that you usually enjoy. When the days become shorter, SAD generally starts in fall or winter and stays until the happier spring days.

Anxiety

Anxiety is an aspect of all life events, an emotional sensation that is also universal. Its natural function is to alert us to potential threats, analyze them, and react to them accurately. This improved planning will also encourage individuals to increase their productivity and develop creative drives. As a modern social phenomenon, anxiety is often seen and expressed in the arts, music, literature, and social media. Anxiety triggers extreme or exaggerated responses to possible threats, leading to chronic and debilitating symptoms linked to disorganizations of anxiety such as fear, phobia, and repeated behaviors that also undermine the lives of people.

Owing to the stresses of daily life, everyone feels anxiety. It is not rare. Feeling overwhelmed at a certain level is inevitable in our fast-paced, complicated, and busy times. Before delivering a speech at the workplace or going for a work interview, it is possible to feel anxiety. Before meeting the love of your life or going on a first date, it's also easy to feel nervous.

Anxiety is a pretty common phenomenon required for the survival of the human race, contrary to popular opinion. The senses of early humans developed to follow a method of raising alarms that triggered an urgent call to action due to the presence of danger from predators, climate conditions, and environmental hazards. Adrenaline streamed through the bloodstream, preparing the body for a response to flight or battle. Adrenaline spikes are typically related to increased sensitivity, increased heart rate, and sweating. The development of human society has diminished the fear of danger from predators in recent times. We also experience anxiety from various sources in today's world, such as family, jobs, well-being, finance, social life, etcetera. A direct manifestation of the flight or battle response is the nervousness that dawns on us before a critical appointment like an interview or meeting.

In psychology, anxiety is used as a general term to describe concern, anticipation, nervousness, and fear. These feelings in daily life are very commonplace to encounter. Still, as they begin to obstruct a human's life, they appear to increase in intensity. Extreme anxiety can contribute to physical symptoms requiring clinical assistance.

Symptoms and Signs of Anxiety

Too much sweat, getting sleepy, loss of focus, restlessness, lack of sleep, elevated heartbeat, and rapid breathing are general signs. Symptoms of anxiety are different among people, so they will all have other symptoms. However, there is no exact reason for anxiety since it mostly depends on one's environment and biology as well.

Anxiety is the defensive response of the body when a threat is perceived. The signs and symptoms of anxiety can be classified into three main categories outlined below:

When a threat is perceived, anxiety is the body's defense response. The signs and symptoms of anxiety can be grouped into the following three major categories:

Physical signs:

- Fast respiration

- Hot flushes

- Tightness in the chest

- Heart rate racing

Psychological symptoms:

- Fear

- Catastrophizing

- Worrying

- Overthinking

Aside from these main classifications, there are other common symptoms of anxiety. They include the following:

- Weakness

- High blood pressure

- Restlessness

- Twitching in muscles

- Lethargic reactions

- Nervousness

- Digestive complications

- Heavy perspiration

- Insomnia

- Feelings of dread or panic

Types of Anxiety

There are different kinds of anxiety in the world today, but in this section, we will only consider some of them:

General Anxiety Disorder

The most common of all is this type of anxiety and is widely known by the acronym GAD. Most of the time, people with general anxiety disorder tend to experience feelings of worry and anxiety. It is like a state of anxiety and nervousness that never dissipates and happens without any known causes. Alternatively, elements that would not usually contribute to anxiety may also cause it. GAD is usually related to symptoms such as restlessness, pessimistic thought, difficulty with concentrating, lethargy, exhaustion, decreased energy levels, among others.

Social Anxiety

Social anxiety is both irrational and inexplicable, referring to any form of fear surrounding social situations. Although some measure of shyness in public situations tends to be a natural occurrence, when it comes to social situations such as public speaking, meeting strangers or power figures, et cetera, people with this form of anxiety usually experience emotions of anxiety and fear. Socializing is a distressing indulgence for people with this type of anxiety. Typically, their anxiety derives from the fear of being rejected, judged, or spoken ill of. Such worries lead them to stay away from social circumstances.

Panic Disorder

A significant cause of worry and terror, capable of having physical and mental consequences, is panic disorder. Physically and psychologically, the symptoms of panic disorders show themselves. They appear to become so severe that hospitalization can result. Increased heart rate, chest pain, profuse sweating, digestive problems, light-headedness, or dizziness are common signs of panic attacks. People with this type of anxiety, along with all these symptoms, often appear to experience feelings of doom, helplessness, and anxiety.

Anxiety and depression are distinct from individuals. The sensations in the stomach can range from getting butterflies. You can also feel like what is happening in your body is no longer out of control. Between the wits and the body, there will be a disconnection. Some individuals can have nightmares, have a sense of fear, and even have traumatic thoughts or memories that you can't manage. Some may worry about locations or events or get worried.

It can also be a very challenging emotion to control anxiety and depression. The world does, after all, have so many stressors. I made this book because I want you to know that anxiety is a natural emotion, that you are not alone, and that you have the power and capacity to cope with it.

Effects of Covid-19 to Mental Health and How to Overcome Them

Mental health problems are spreading along with it as Coronavirus spreads globally. Even though we are all experiencing this situation, which can cause trauma, it is also important to note that different issues are more prevalent for other people.

The lockdown may be a moment for contemplation for some of us, and it may be a time of intense stress and suffering for some. Some of us may face intense loneliness, violence, financial difficulties, or health scares, and some of us may not. It doesn't mean that anyone's experience is right or wrong; this variety is just necessary to note. We all cope differently with this lockout and often feel varying levels of tension and anxiety.

The name itself causes fear of unknowingness, tension, and anxiety-Corona Virus Disease. It has caused a dramatic loss of human life worldwide and has impacted many others' well-being. Add to this the massive economic loss and social disruption, which is devastating.

Many firms have shut down, and many face existential challenges. It affects employment directly. Many lose work, and many got pay cuts. Their monthly expense plans are directly affected by this. People struggle to pay EMIs, rents, medical expenses, and other expenses under stress. Family members burdened whose breadwinner has lost jobs or lost to Covid-19 infection. Words are not adequate to describe their emotional disruption. Their tears say their secret tale!

We've seen how, internationally, the corona pandemic induces tension and anxiety. What is the next move, then? For an extended period, we cannot cope with this tension and anxiety. So, it's time for a solution for the next move!

The "Super 6" formula is a simple formula that not only allows you to de-stress and relax during the pandemic crisis but also for your whole life. Bear in mind that everything you do to stay stress-free has a direct positive influence on your family. You get upset with little stuff when you are nervous and depressed, and you over-react. It affects your family directly, as well as your interpersonal relationship. By the same reasoning, if you stay stress-free, calm, and satisfied, you naturally display understanding when interacting with family members and thus positively impact your interpersonal relationship.

## 1.	Reduce Stressors

A stressor, what is it? In simple language, a stressor is called something that creates stress in you. The current pandemic of Covid-19 has produced extreme stress that affects all of us worldwide. In the current pandemic, the most critical stressors include:

- Fear of coronavirus infection

- Fear of losing the job

- Financial loss in the organization

- A weakening economy that damages companies

- Elderly or other family members' health problems that could cause financial expenses

- Declining bank savings as used for everyday needs (groceries, drugs, milk, etc.) without revenue inflow due to lockdown or loss of jobs

- Stress if a member of the family got infected with Covid-19

- Death of nearby people due to Covid19

- Isolation or time of quarantine

- Practicing social isolation

The above stressors cause stress and affect our physical health, mental health, and psychological health, which, in turn, affects our behavior.

To avoid these, you could do the following:

• As you have learned about the social distance to keep our protection from coronavirus infection. Along with social distancing, to keep your mind healthy from being poisoned by stress and anxiety, you will need to practice social media distancing.

• Stop too much conversation with family, colleagues, etc., about pandemic subjects. The more you speak, the more anxiety is produced inside you.

• Often affirm optimistic statements such as "The world is safe", "The universe is safe and well cared for by my family and me," "I am financially stable," etc. You can even make an affirmation of your own.

2.   Positive Thinking

Good thought impacts us positively. Let us see only a few advantages of positive thinking.

Positive Thinking Benefits:

- Improved immune system

- Reduced levels of tension

- Reduces the chances of depression significantly

- Greater tolerance to mainstream cold

- Psychological well-being improved

- Enhanced physical health and mental health

- Enhanced relationships for everyone

- Cardio-vascular system healthy

- Plainness of thought-process

- Optimistic approach to unfavorable circumstances

- Helps to trust your skills

• Most significantly, individuals would love to be your friend and companion! You'll find that many of us strive to stop negative-thinking individuals.

3. Spend Time with Your Family

The most significant part and the cornerstone of our lives is family life. Family time is the greatest stress buster on this planet and the best relief treatment! It helps to improve emotional bonding as well.

All were busy running after career, job, worldly pleasures, social media life, friend circle, etc., until the recent corona outbreak. It left so little time for the family to spend. I saw many people returning from work, having dinner, and then spending hours on social media. The virtual world has become so much like our real world that we can't even remember the last time we spoke to our true mates. A lot of people have thousands of virtual friends, but not even 25 real friends! Thousands of social media fans, but not even five real-world followers!

Due to the Covid-19 pandemic, lockdown gave us a chance to step back and look back at our mistakes. It is time to rectify our errors. Few spend unnecessary time on social media, mobile phones, TV, etc., even during the lockdown, rather than spending this quality time with family. There is no question that the world of social media has its meaning and significance, but a balance is required.

Let us understand the meaning of life as a family. The moment we are born, our family's warmth, mainly father and mother, embraces us. We are brought up with our parents' warmth. As we grow and go out, with different mindsets and different upbringing, we meet different people. We also get hurt emotionally during this outer world contact. But we feel light and content being with our family members when we are back home because they are our first universe. We're feeling safe. Isn't that an excellent stress-buster? Just imagine the last time it began to rain heavily, or there was a cyclone, or the roads were chaotic. The first thing that came to mind then was how easily I would be able to reach home. We were under stress and anxiety before we got home. And we were feeling an unknown fear as well. But the moment we walked home, we felt a rush of lightness and happiness, and we felt safe and happy. Why are we at home feeling safe and secure? As our family is with us!

For the sake of fleeting gratification, though, we prefer to waste too much time with friends in the virtual world, social media, and unnecessary time. So, let's change our old habits today and get into a new routine where we spend quality time with family and build family values while juggling our world of social media, friendship, and career. Take some time with your family to laugh!

4.   Integrated Self-Detox

We all recognize that heavy intake of fast food, alcohol, smoking, low-fiber food, etc., creates toxins in the body over some time. We exercise to eliminate these toxins, increase water intake, take vitamins, increase fruit and green leafy vegetables, etc. It is to rid our physical body of contaminants and refer to physical body detox. But that is not adequate. What about clearing pollutants at the level of mind and emotion?

We need to detox in the modern-day lifestyle and particularly during this corona pandemic:

- Physical body

- Mental Body

- Emotional Body

I term this as "Integrated Self-Detox."

Self-Detox was also crucial in the past, but because of the corona pandemic crisis and global recession, and economic blast, it has never been as important today.

We will learn how to detox ourselves so that we can maintain good health in all our three bodies - physical body, mental body, and emotional body -. The balance will help us maintain good health in these three bodies and make us feel energetic. Emotional Strength and Inner Peace will help us grow. Imbalance in any one body would have negative effects on the other two bodies.

Self-detoxing is very easy. Remember, it all starts with "I". Some family members see modifications in me as "I" self-detox. They will get inspired to keep following you when they see changes in you. They'll be keen on self-detoxification.

In this stressful time, self-detox is currently truly relevant as we bear fear, anxiety, and stress of covid19, global recession, the effect of cash flow, anxiety due to social isolation, quarantine, fear of another lockout, fear of losing jobs, etc. Because of this, our brain and body are frequently under stress. Stress impairs the activity of our glands, nervous system, parasympathetic nervous system, and organs. Stress is like a poison that's sluggish.

So, let us get ready for Self-Detox Incorporated. It's important to remember that it should be part of your everyday lifestyle. It will become so ingrained in you over some time that it automatically becomes part of your lifestyle and daily routine.

5.   Stay Updated

Because of this pandemic of the corona, many are going out of business. To thrive, many organizations that have used conventional approaches need to adjust. Today, the digital world has become the new standard. Only people who have updated their skills and expertise will thrive in this time of crisis and the coming years. Some of you will need to change your business model to survive.

Self-Update is your survival key. For entrepreneurs, Self-Update requires a business model and business strategies, not just skills and experience. And this refers to the latest global pandemic, as well as after the conclusion of the pandemic. And by the time the pandemic is over, the world will change the way corporations do. In the next 2-3 years, a lot of changes will happen. We need to prepare ourselves so that we can survive.

Regardless of the global heat of the crisis, the performance slogan for all of us is to stay "updated." And it extends to all fields of professional services and industry.

6.   Gratitude

Gratitude provides greater satisfaction in positive psychology studies. Research has shown that gratitude allows individuals to have more positive feelings that enhance their health, boost the immune system, feel alive and have compassion.

People can use gratitude in many aspects of your life, including company, relationship, parents, schooling, career, work, finances, friends, etc.

How Depression and Anxiety Affects Relationships

In intimate relationships, nervous feelings exacerbate. An anxious person struggles with unresolved worries and fears. While this unique condition has been distinguished from other anxiety conditions by the Diagnostic and Statistical Manual and put on a trauma scale, the trauma that may cause PTSD **(Posttraumatic stress disorder)** is not different from the causes facing anxious individuals.

An anxious person may respond more strongly to interaction than someone who does not suffer from excessive worry. What causes the sufferer to feel nervous is that it is not always easy to tease out a valid concern and an unreasonable or dysfunctional concern. Think of someone with PTSD **(Posttraumatic stress disorder)** being the case. An individual engaged in battle is likely to attach importance to loud noises, the sight of weapons, or confrontation to the degree that someone who has not engaged in combat has. It doesn't mean that adding sense to this stuff is incorrect, but they are more held in them than everyone else has.

Although there is no general cause for concern, people with anxiety can appear to have extreme reactions to situations in a way that seems excessive, just as if in the past they had undergone trauma. Some psychologists think that anxiety may be more prevalent in individuals who have experienced trauma, but this theory does not entirely account for anxiety prevalence. Conditions of anxiety are shown to be more commonplace in Western countries, in women, and in families, too. In the sense of trauma, it is not easy to clarify any of this, but a clear rule for someone unfamiliar with anxiety would be to treat distressed men and women as though they were subject to trauma.

This approach aims not to marginalize or view anxious people in some fundamental way as abnormal. Instead, the point is to make the reader feel sympathy for the anxious person. Compassion involves recognizing what the other person is going through and having a degree of empathy and tolerance for what they are going through. It can be difficult for someone who is not anxious to realize what it feels like to have ongoing problems.

Thinking of anxious individuals as being more keyed into or words and behavior is about more than compassionate. This method also encourages the person to be aware of what they say and do that could cause or exacerbate the anxious person's response. Just like you may avoid playing a noisy rap song full of gunshot sounds in front of a person with PTSD **(Posttraumatic stress disorder)** or avoid taking them to a party full of people, flashing lights, and garnish sounds. Similarly, you can avoid the things that can exacerbate your significant other's anxiety.

An anxious person may have a propensity to overanalyze, adding significance to items that to you may seem trivial. You may suggest doing this or that, or you may even have a long list of possibilities. You can suggest, or even have a long list of options, to do this or that. When dealing with an anxious person, this may not be the best approach because they may obsess about all the facets of the choices you have given them rather than concentrate on only one issue.

Having the Right Approach to Anxiety in a Relationship

Some psychologists suggest that the negative connotations that some people who do not have anxiety can attach to anxiety can make anxiety worse for the significant other, making the experience of coping with anxiousness worse for all individuals in the relationship. These psychiatrists have written a lot about the possibility that maybe knowing it and being curious about it is the best way to coping with anxiety in the relationship setting. From the perspective of fear, approaching anxiety raises the probability of a negative interaction since you project your preconceived concepts onto the interaction.

Maybe it helps to think like this about it. We live in an age of information. This age of knowledge we live in can be a good thing, but it can be a negative thing. Getting access to information helps us educate ourselves on a wide range of subjects with the click of a mouse or a finger's swipe. Today, data of a comprehensive nature is easier to access than it was in the past. But that is just one aspect of the age of information. Another result of this social transition is that people can now engage with each other in ways they have not been able to before.

It is an era of instant contact, truly. You can use this immediate contact for good or not. In a moment, this will all become apparent. Let us presume that someone in the group wishes to go to a nearby restaurant. For whatever reason, this person (or couple) has a bad experience. Maybe the waiter was a little short, maybe the food was cold, or maybe the food wasn't to their liking. This person (or couple) then uses social media to talk about their bad experiences to everyone. Others will now either completely avoid the restaurant or be likely to see their own potential experience negatively.

But if you were to go to the restaurant from the perspective of curiosity, rather than with your preconceived ideas about the restaurant, then maybe your experience would be different. You may have regularly walked by the restaurant before the bad review and noticed all the happy people sitting inside or coming out of the restaurant. Perhaps the restaurant serves cuisine that you are especially fond of. Instead of going to the restaurant with the idea of confirming the bad ideas you've learned, maybe eating there with curiosity is the better approach: satisfying a long interest in eating in this particular establishment.

Don't approach anxious people (or a specific anxious person) with preconceived notions based on stories you have heard. Perhaps you have learned that a specific individual is "difficult" (or whatever not particularly nice word people choose to refer to someone else that they do not like). Instead of assuming that what you have learned is accurate (and it might not be very good) and using that data to direct your relationship with the person, you might keep an open mind. Maybe it was the other person who was difficult, and the anxious person only reacted in a dysfunctional way to another person. You never fully understand that the experiences and opinions you learn from others are accurate. It's always a good idea to have an open mind about stuff like this when it comes to mental health conditions.

This approach to anxiety not only helps you to have a stronger response than you would otherwise have, but it also enables you to be the caring, considerate human being you can be (and that you want to be). You're not reading this book because you're someone who lacks empathy, and your goal is to be as inconsiderate as possible to anxious individuals. If you are reading this book, it is either because there is someone in your life who struggles from concern and wants to be more conscious of, or because you have the situation yourself. You are interested in how you can handle the pitfalls that come with being in a relationship.

Both partnerships are rife with pitfalls. It is just as true for relationships where one party has a mental health disorder for relationships where both partners are ostensibly "normal" individuals. They claim that no one is truly "normal" can, of course, be made. Society decides what is normal, and the men and women who are members of that society are all striving to fulfill the normal social notion. This knowledge of the almost arbitrary essence of normalcy, if anything, should encourage you to be a little more compassionate to anxious people or those who are undergoing their mental health problems.

Therefore, when it comes to maintaining a relationship with someone with anxiety, the best thing to consider is to be curious about their symptoms and desire to learn more. It will help you approach the relationship from the perspective of learning more about the other person. That possibly drew them to you-rather than embarking on this path with ideas based on minimal understanding, gossip, and the like about the other person.

A significant piece of advice that psychotherapists sometimes say to their clients as a coping mechanism is the second thing to note. Around the globe, men and women are all struggling with their troubles. You don't know what they might be dealing with in their lives when you meet someone, which can make life more complicated for them. It can, of course, be a challenge to always understand others' internal states, particularly when others can, sadly, not understand our inner conditions. But we can distinguish between the dysfunction that others encounter and the possible dysfunction that we may infuse into our own lives by understanding that others have their internal emotional states and challenges and that our emotional states are different.

That's just an introduction to the advice offered by psychotherapists; we've not yet gotten to the significant bit. So, what's the direction that psychiatrists offer as a coping mechanism to their patients? You should not let the emotional state of another person determine your own. It is not clear advice given explicitly for coping with people with anxiety. Indeed, this is general advice to navigate life in a world that might seem to be going off the deep end more and more. It is a way for you to preserve your sanity.

This piece of advice is getting at because you should not allow the frustration, sorrow, rage, or other reactionary emotion of another person to affect how you feel and behave. It is not to suggest that nervous people always have negative feelings and inspire negative emotions while this can often happen. The idea here is that your mental state is different from that of the person you are dealing with, so you need to be able to say, "This individual is not angry for whatever reason, and I'm all right with that." For me, there is no need to get angry.

What this does is, even in the sense of dealing with someone who might be frustrated, concerned, or otherwise upset, it helps you to stay calm and free of worries. It can be easy to respond to others' emotional states by being as emotional as they are. It is a kind of defensive mechanism. In fact, in individuals who have anxiety, depression, a personality disorder, or any condition that affects how the individual views the world and communicates with it, this form of strategy may be more regular.

Anxious people tend, in other words, to react to things in unstable ways. They can interpret things you say and do as dangerous, complicated, aggressive, or in different ways that their brain interprets as not benign. The last thing you need to do is to respond similarly to their emotional response. If you learn that you've upset them with everything you've said or done, it's not helpful for someone to upset you too. One thing you can do, which is the best, is to understand that the other person is upset for some reason and then recognize that you are not sore and there is no reason for you to become bitter.

This approach achieves several things. The first thing it does is that by reacting in kind, it saves you from worsening the other person's fear or emotion. If your partner is angry, it won't make matters any better if you get upset. The second thing that this strategy does is ultimately diffuses a crisis (in most cases). If you stay calm and project an image of serenity and happiness, this may indicate that things are all right for the anxious individual and that there is no reason for them to be defensive.

Of course, by always being the one who stays calm, it is not easy to always be the person that reacts to anger, hostility, or some other emotional reaction. As you are the one who is still supposed to be calm and level-headed when the other person is a screaming psycho, you may begin to feel like you are being taken advantage of. But here, it is essential to note that an anxious or traumatized person tends to respond to uncertain or unfamiliar circumstances defensively or emotionally. In other words, if you apply this tactic of staying calm in front of another person long enough, that person can ultimately see that you are not threatening (and the little things you do) and that they do not need to respond defensively to you.

10 Easy Ways to Overcome Anxiety and Depression

1.   Smile More Often

Did do ever hear that a smile is one of the best presents to give a person? It is so real. Smiling doesn't cost you anything. It gives you a shiny, inviting outlook instead.

The latest research has shown that smiling has a fantastic way of improving one's mood. What lessons are there to learn?

Smile frequently. If it doesn't come naturally to you, begin first by pushing it. Think of a funny incident or acts in the past as you carry out your everyday tasks, then create a smile from there. You will learn the art over time, and it will come naturally in your daily life. So, what are the places where you can smile? There is no specific rule, but these will help:

•   At your workplace

•   When someone walks past you

- While at home

- During a phone conversation

Something to Try: After reading this part, find a person to smile!

2.   Don't Dwell on Negative Thoughts.

Negativity has a way of consuming you entirely. From the present moment, it takes you away. Unfortunately, many people waste unnecessary time focusing on negative thoughts for days, weeks, or even months. But, in a situation where you find yourself in a fix, what can you do?

Drive negative feelings further. Pause and focus on whether that thinking benefits you for a moment; you'll undoubtedly remember it doesn't. Then think of a worthwhile thing: something that would lift your mood.

3.   Show How Grateful You Are for What You Have

Not only are you expected to be thankful for what you have, but you can also prove it.

When something good happens, it is easy to be positive, but it is always more challenging to reflect on the things you are thankful for when hard times arise. You will feel happier during these periods by reflecting on your situation's good aspects or by thinking about positive memories of your life to avoid negative thoughts. What should you be grateful for? Your circumstances depend on it. But here are some things for which you should be thankful:

- Family

- Friends

- Your Job

- Good Memories

- Opportunities

- Being Alive

So, don't forget to think about things you are thankful for during a tumultuous time.

4. Stay Bright in Each Bad Experience

It's been said that there are right sides to any poor situation. For example, someone has an accident: he/she loses his/her expensive smartphone or his/her assets, potentially the debtor's fund that he or she owes. Yeah, that's an unfortunate event, but is that all he/she can think of?

He should be thankful for the fact that he/she is safe and alive! Also, constructive thinking helps you to translate negative experiences into life lessons, allowing you to recognize your mistakes and prevent you from twice making the same ones.

In this way, if you learn to do things better each time, you will be able to prevent any negative experiences or be well prepared if a similar occurrence happens in the future.

5.   Spend Quality Time with positive-minded Individuals

There are various theories and philosophies that many individuals bring about. Others are good and hopeful thoughts, while others are bad and pessimistic thoughts. Those who think negatively are likely to attract mates with similar thought habits, whereas positive-minded people are also likely to attract individuals who think similarly. Birds of a feather flock together, after all.

Cutting off negative friends could be helpful; that means spending less time with them and seeking out other, more positive people like yourself. Thus, optimistic thoughts will accompany you.

You feel bad and are more likely to suffer from low self-esteem if you spend more time with negative people; on the flip side, spending time with more positive people will help you feel better about yourself!

6. Calm Your Mind

It may be a unique ability that takes commitment, consistency, and patience to relax your mind. The reason why quieting your mind is advantageous is that having peace in yourself has several advantages. Once you find peace on the inside, with any situation and circumstance you surround yourself with, it will become simpler to pursue peace outside of you. The inner peace mind's goal isn't to prevent thinking but to surpass the barriers that the mind keeps you trapped in.

7. Consciously and purposely challenge your thoughts

Cognitive-behavioral therapy revolves around this approach. Many psychologists swear by this approach because it ensures that you can regulate or shift your thoughts and establish new patterns or behaviors of communicating with your thoughts in a particular way. By confronting them, you retake power. Begin by telling yourself about your ideas. If your feeling is that you're just not all right, then ask yourself where it comes from. Are you jumping to conclusions? Which one does this thought fall under among the cognitive distortions? It will provide the perspective to take back your power to find the source of the thinking and where it comes from, and you will then substitute it with reality.

8. Intentionally specialize in your breathing

Often, we get anxious, worried, or depart our "false alarm" triggers because we aren't breathing properly. Close your eyes and specialize in whether your breath is coming from your stomach, chest, or nose. Next, without altering it, practice feeling your pulse. You will then specialize in taking deep, long breaths until you have figured out where your breath is coming from and the way you breathe. Count on inhaling for 5 seconds, holding for 3 seconds, and exhaling for 5 to 7 seconds. Repeat until you feel calmer, and then, before opening your eyes again, return to normal breathing.

9.   **Play calming music that relaxes and motivates you**

One of the simplest healers out there is music. They'll become our favorite artists once we can relate to the singer, and then we'll feel more relaxed knowing they're singing about something that means something to you. If your thing is more instrumental, focus on the rhythm and, therefore, the instruments' noise. Close your eyes and try to hear sounds from a distance that you have never heard before. Try to recall the devices and memorize the melody.

10.   **Participate in regular exercise**

It releases those "feel good" chemicals when we exercise daily. It becomes more straightforward for our brains to supply more serotonin when dopamine is released, which helps us feel happy. We don't feel so anxious once we are content, and our emotions aren't as overwhelming or overpowering. The goal is to physically figure out our bodies so our minds don't have the energy to overthink or generate mental chatter. Mental chatter gets worse when we overthink, stress unnecessarily, or think all the time negatively, and it may seem not easy to fix it. On the road to rebooting the brain, I will be able to explore strategies.

The Role of Nature and Support from Loved Ones

Once you are ready, you are going to need support. You are going to need to tell people about your plan. It should not be your little kept secret. If your addiction has been a secret, then this is the time for you to tell everyone of it.

The reason you need to tell people is not that you need them to know you have been taking painkillers to get through each day. It's not because you need to be accountable for what you have been doing. You need to tell people that you need to be responsible for what you are going to do. It will help if you let as many people as you can in on your venture of quitting opiates.

Tell the right people – the people who will be supportive of you. Tell the people who will be excited for you and who will show it on their faces. Tell the people who are going to cheer you on. Tell the people who are not afraid to ask you how your sobriety is going later. Ask them to ask you about your gravity later.

One of the most important things that a spouse or partner of an anxious person has to recognize is that their role in the process is as a supporter. It may be the case that you know your significant other better than anyone else, but that still leaves the task of dealing with anxiousness primarily to them rather than to you.

The role of the supporter is an important one. This chapter aims to provide you with tips that you can use to help you fulfill this role in the best way you can. Sure, sitting on the sidelines can be frustrating sometimes, but a solid supporter is just what your partner or spouse needs right now. And if you are dealing with anxiousness, then these tips will help you understand the sorts of things that your partner can do for you.

1. **Do not be judgmental.**

This first tip may be a no-brainer to some readers. But it is not a no-brainer for everyone, which is why it is essential to mention it here. Depression and anxiety are not easy to deal with, including the depressed person himself or herself. One of the reasons why there is so much stigma surrounding depression and anxiety is that many people have preconceived notions about depression. These notions may come from perceptions they have about depressed people they have seen or misconceptions about why a particular person is depressed.

"Snap out of it" is something that someone may be inclined to say to a depressed person. A statement like this might have been perfectly reasonable to speak to someone whc is depressed in the past. Still, now we understand that depression stems ultimately from disorders in brain chemistry, so the individual may not be able to snap out of it. Perhaps the first practical step you can take

53

toward supporting someone who is depressed is deciding not to be judgmental. Depressive illness is hard. This condition looks different in different people, and depression does not go away when we project our negative judgments onto depressed people.

2. **Educate yourself about depression and anxiety first, before you plan your "strike."**

In reality, you, the reader, have taken one of the most significant first steps in supporting someone with sadness. Men and women are often judgmental about depressed people because they do not know much about depression. A person who has never experienced depression is sure to have a host of preconceived notions that impact how they perceive depressed people that they meet, even when that person is someone close to them like a partner or spouse.

Therefore, before you even begin to think of a "plan of attack" in dealing with sadness in a significant other, you need first to make sure that you have an understanding of depression. It would be best if you understood what depression is, what some of the causes of depression are, what the warning signs are, and how sadness can drastically impact the lives of depressed people and those around them. You would not be reading this book if you did not have some interest in educating yourself on the subject so let the education continue.

3. Understand that overcoming anxiety and depression is a process.

Anxiety is not like having a common cold. It is not something that you get and which you will experience resolution from with a finger's snap. Anxiety disorders should be thought of as conditions that require treatment. It means that you should be realistic about your partner's anxiety for the significant other of an anxious person. They will not snap out of their anxiety, and it is more than a little unfair of you to expect them. As a supporter of an anxious person, it is critical to recognize that you will be helping them through the long process of overcoming their illness.

4. Be conscious of your dysfunctional thoughts or preconceived notions.

Anxiousness is characterized by a cavalcade of dysfunctional thoughts that people often are not conscious of. Unfortunately for the significant others of anxious persons, they can spiral dysfunctional beliefs that can impact how they perceive and interact with their anxious partner. It's not that the partner is necessarily at risk for worry, but merely that the partner should recognize how notions can color their interaction (including the subconscious stigma that men and women often have towards needs of the mind).

5. Provide reassurance that things are going to turn out all right.

One of the most important things that someone is supporting someone else through anxiety (or any condition) can provide reassurance that things are going to turn out all right. It does not mean telling a lie. If someone has a terminal illness like stage IV cancer, it is vital to recognize what that means. But honest reassurance in the case of anxiousness is a little different. Anxiety can and does frequently get better, so reminding your partner of that can place a positive thought in their head that can be an essential part of creating real change in their life.

6. Encourage your partner to get help.

A complicated reality for some partners of anxious people to accept is that it is not their job to steer their partner they think they should go. We have established that anxiety disorders typically do not get better without treatment, but you can't force them to get treatment or dictate to them the form that the treatment should take.

Intervention-type maneuvers can be problematic in mental health. It is especially true in the case of anxiousness, where the individual may already be inclined to have a suspicious or fearful approach to others or the world in general. Forcing or cornering your partner into treatment is not a good idea for anxious people. You can educate yourself about the help that is available for their condition and encourage them to get help. That is all that you can do.

7. Be patient as your significant other moves through their condition.

It is essential to be patient when dealing with a person with a mental health condition, which is just as accurate of anxiety as other conditions like depression. Recall that anxiety disorders include conditions as divergent as GAD, specific phobias, and obsessive-compulsive disorder. The point here is that some of these conditions can be very debilitating for the individual dealing with and very frustrating for the partner or family member who is around it. For your sanity (and for the sake of your partner), it is essential to be patient. The change will happen slowly, and it will help you to keep this in mind.

8. **Avoid the aggressive, interventional approach.**

It is easy to see depression as something dysfunctional in another person's life that needs to go away. There are television shows that involve handling dysfunction from what can be thought of as an intervention or interventional approach. In the context of depression, it means pouncing or cornering the depressed person (often with other family and loved ones involved) to impress the person how bad their condition has been to themselves and their people.

Although this approach may be useful in people with substance abuse disorders, it probably is not the best approach for dealing with anxiety. Your significant other should be someone that you trust and who trusts you. They most likely are looking to you as someone they can go to for support, and they may be waiting for the opportunity to broach the subject of depression with you if they have not already. Confronting them angrily or forcefully with their depression is not necessary, and it is potentially damaging.

9. Use simple gestures to show that you care.

Although some readers may approach this book as a weapon in their arsenal to declaring war on depression and winning that action, in reality, a depressed person may need to know that you care. Although the war analogy may be apt for the subject of depression, when it comes to supporting someone who is depressed, it might be better to think of depression as an illness. Someone who is suffering from a disease does not want to be attacked or confronted.

Sure, you may feel that as you are not depressed, you are perfectly poised to help your depressed partner, but you have to recognize that they are doing things on their own time and have a right. As much as you may want this depression to go away now, it may be that the individual needs some time to come to grips with their depression and formulate a way of dealing with it. In this regard, depression maybe likes the grieving process. It is something that people go through, and what they may need during this time is a kind word, a card, or some gesture that indicates that you care.

10. Do not project your perceptions and experiences onto the other person.

Depression is a subjective experience. That is one of the fascinating things about it. Even though we can say that depressive illness results from a chemical imbalance, we have to recognize that each depressed person is a unique person with their unique set of thoughts and experiences.

What that means for you is that even if you educate yourself about this condition, there will still be aspects of your significant other's subjective experience of depression closed off to you. Just as you have elements of yourself that other people do not understand, so too does your partner has parts of him or herself that you do not understand. This tip is related to the direction of not being judgmental, although it is not the same. You have to be careful as a loving partner not to project your perceptions of depression and why they may be depressed onto your partner. The goal here is not to be Dr. Freud but to be an influential supporter.

It applies to partners and can even be helpful for family members or even just friends. Do not neglect someone just because they have depression and anxiety. Be a supporter and do your role well.

I Have Overcome It, and So Can You

I, myself, have experienced anxiety and depression. I have gone through that phase in my life as well. I have been for five years. Do not be afraid because, just like me, you will eventually overcome it. It takes time, but you will get there.

What comes to mind when you hear anxiety? Is it someone that's fretful, disheveled, and talking rapidly? While those certainly are signs of an anxious person, there are also more subtle signs that most people either don't recognize or downplay. For example, when standing in line to pay a bill, do you find yourself breathing erratically? What about when the light turns red when you realize you are late for work or an appointment? Don't mislabel people as impatient or irritable; the truth is the impatience and irritability are symptoms. The source is anxiety, to some degree or the other, and it's anxiety that has put millions of people on the road to a high tense lifestyle full of disappointments and frustrations. There is hope, even if you've struggled with anxiety for years. I was determined to control it (and depression) instead of those demons controlling me.

The cousin to anxiety is depression; although anxiety is mostly circumstantial, depression goes deeper than that. Far more profound, and if the two are encountered continuously without a practical system to manage them, the victim can suffer a life beyond misery. Depression serves no fair use; its long-reaching effects are never positive (unless used to learn by and build a positive system to manage it). Depression is rooted in darkness, whereas anxiety is the high-energy counterpart; each alone is a formidable opponent but combined, they are tough to overcome. The good news is there are ways to pick each apart and learn what it is and how it operates then once the first is manageable, attack on the second. Yes, attacked, these ailments don't play nice; they seek to destroy. Some will argue that point, but the truth remains, show me somebody that has ever truly benefited from being an anxious, depressed person exactly.

I know firsthand what anxiety and depression are, and I see the environment where anxiety, depression, panic attacks, hatred, anger, and a whole host of mental disorders breeds. I know pain, the pain only God saw me go through, and the pain that has no words to describe it. I know what it feels like to sweat and shake like a damned rag doll over going into a social situation that most people feel is nothing at all to even think about. I know depression and how it feels to want to die every day you exist; I know how it feels about planning out your suicide and that dark place you live in when depression takes over your mind. I know.

For years I thought that my anxiety and depression were unmanageable, and I accepted them as part of who I was. I had no idea that these ailments could be changed or managed. But the power of gratitude and laughter therapy helped me to get over it.

Practice gratitude to enjoy the fullness of life. When you are grateful, the negatives turn to positives; the chaos becomes in order, and confusion converts to clarity. It is only possible by having a grateful attitude. By doing this, you fill your mind with gratitude and create a happier you.

It is not that everything in your life is harmful and is against you. The situation that you are facing is only in a section of your life. Therefore, it is good to appreciate what you have in life. It is good, to begin with, your own life; you are going through tough times, but God has given you a chance to live. It is a reason to show gratitude. One can also cultivate gratitude by engaging in charity work such as helping those who are less fortunate, such as the poor, old, children living in children's homes, and street children. This gesture can make one feel good about themselves and start appreciating and loving their lives.

The person realizes that he is the right person and deserves fair treatment and a better life. I thank God that he has given me good health, and why should I languish in depression, and yet some people do not have what I have. Gratitude arouses such questions, which brings out positivity, and encourages focus. The person with such an awakening force will align his or her action towards healing from depression. He or she now feels obligated to make his life better. The new energy is right to fight the emotions that cause changes in mood and anxiety.

Laughter therapy also helped me a lot. Humor is highly subjective—what brings giggles to one person could get another to sleep just as quickly. Part of laughter therapy is to find out just what the funny bone tickles because it can be as easy as tossing in a DVD to get some healing laughs. Have no doubt, though, of dealing with a curmudgeon who disregards Woody Allen's wit or those madcap Muppets.

Laughter therapy advocates don't just limit themselves to jokes.

Fake laughter, similar to real laughter, can be useful. It includes a laughter coach who will implore you to pretend that your arms are paws and roar with laughter. Or maybe you'll be invited to do some lawnmower laughter, acting to start a mower with a couple of warm-up chuckles, eventually turning to a full laugh. People who lead laughter therapy sessions have discovered that the real kind usually gives way to these fake laughs.

To figure out what makes you happy and maintain the ability in daily situations to find humor will alleviate the stress and anxiety that comes with the challenges of life. You can choose to be a horrible depression and sink it. You will have more resources to fight by deciding to laugh and promote happiness. It holds for everything from sickness to an assignment to dealing with your worst nemesis—if you find ways to laugh, you stay in charge, even if everything else appears to be out of your hands.

Dealing with depression is tricky; it varies so much from one person to the next. Anxiety does the same, but there are more generalized patterns and traits that are recognizable with depression. Both ailments originate nearby and operate in the same domain, but their triggers can differ.

So, you may be asking, what's the point of this story? It's to help others know that I lived what I'm talking about, the depression, the anxiety, the mental hell. I can see those interconnected bridges and see how my life became what it was through my choices and methods to control and manage the battles in my head. I hope that the content in this book can help others recover from these situations.

Conclusion

I will end this book with a few words of hope and encouragement from my experience. I'm alive today; that's the cold hard fact. If you knew how many times I should have 'checked out' of this life, from my fault or not, it's mind-blowing to see me still here. But I am, and so are you. I almost buckled from too much mental anguish and the inability to get a grasp on it.

If I could get all those nights back where I laid awake with anxiety driving my thoughts to the point I seriously thought I was about to go insane or the sleepless nights due to the depression pushing me to the brink of shoving a handgun in my mouth. If I could get all of those moments back and redo them with the knowledge and fortitude I have now, I'd get about many years. If I could take all the pain, the tears that flooded from my eyes, the screams to God, the loneliness, the sadness, the panic attacks that damaged my body, I'd have a new life to live.

Dear reader, please know mental disorders have seasons, just like the law of nature. The sun will come out again; the light will come forth after darkness after suffering comes peace. Please don't give up on finding that peace; never settles for what society tells you about your mental challenges; you are the only one that knows your body, and it's you that owns your body.

Do the work, keep hope alive, love, find beauty in every day and every breath. Learn to live again by managing your anxiety and depression, don't let them control you. I came out alive, and you will too; press on and know others can relate to your struggles and care about you. I wish you the very best, my friend; stay healthy and keep your eyes on the finish line; it's closer than you think!

References:

Dobson, K. S. (1985). The relationship between anxiety and depression. *Clinical Psychology Review*, *5*(4), 307-324.

https://depression.org.nz/is-it-depression-anxiety/anxiety/

https://my.clevelandclinic.org/health/diseases/9536-anxiety-disorders

https://www.medicalnewstoday.com/articles/8933

Stavrakaki, C., & Vargo, B. (1986). The relationship of anxiety and depression: a review of the literature. *The British Journal of Psychiatry*, *149*(1), 7-16.

https://www.yalemedicine.org/news/stress-anxiety-depression

https://highfocuscenters.pyramidhealthcarepa.com/the-relationship-between-depression-and-anxiety/

https://www.nhsinform.scot/illnesses-and-conditions/mental-health/depression

https://www.drugwatch.com/health/mental-health/how-to-deal-with-anxiety/

https://www.depressioncenter.org/toolkit/im-not-feeling-well/learn-about-it/learn-about-depression

https://www.forbes.com/sites/kathycaprino/2020/03/26/how-to-manage-depression-and-anxiety-in-frightening-times/

https://www.ama-assn.org/delivering-care/public-health/why-depression-anxiety-are-prevalent-during-covid-19

Kendall, P. C., & Watson, D. E. (1989). *Anxiety and depression: Distinctive and overlapping features.* Academic Press.

https://www.rtor.org/2019/07/24/how-anxiety-and-depression-affect-your-relationships/

https://studentaffairs.psu.edu/health-wellness/medical-services/health-information-resources/anxiety-depression

https://www.goodrx.com/anxiety/anxiety-and-depression

https://familydoctor.org/condition/depression/